Sheila Granger's Virtual Gastric Band Workbook

The Solution To The Worldwide Obesity Epidemic

Sheila Granger

and

Marc Carlin

Inception House Publishing

Sheila Granger's Virtual Gastric Band Workbook

The Solution To The Worldwide Obesity Epidemic

by Sheila Granger and Marc Carlin

Copyright © 2011 Sheila Granger and Marc Carlin

ISBN: 0-9832785-0-4
ISBN-13: 978-0-9832785-0-4

Inception House Publishing

As a thank you for purchasing this book, I would like to help you along your journey to your desired shape and size with some of the free tools available at:

http://VirtualGastricBandWorkbook.com/bookbonus

You will be able to download a FREE trance recording that will help you practice going into hypnotic trance and begin your journey to change.

Sheila Granger & Marc Carlin

I would like to dedicate this book to my ever supportive family, friends and clients, especially Sonia who is living proof that a person's weight is all in the mind.

~Sheila

Dedicated to my loving and supportive family, Alma, Bryan and Brad, Mom and Dad, and Rochelle and Lori.

~ Marc

CONTENTS

Welcome to the workbook for Sheila Granger's Virtual Gastric Band Program

This program is not a diet. Instead it is a sensible approach that uses a proven method of changing your habitual behavior around food and eating. Diets are designed for failure as their main requirement is the elimination of specific foods and the introduction of new foods. This causes a deprivation mentality and contributes to the diet being a failed exercise in weight loss.

Diets usually fail for a number of reasons - one being that they are episodic, rather like training for a race. For example, if you enter a race, you will begin training prior to the race to condition you body and mind. So if you start training six weeks before the race, planning to finish it and improve your time, you will focus on how you run. You note your speed, distance and pace and as you continue training, over the weeks you work on increasing your speed. All the while you are conditioning yourself to run better and your focus is on the running. During this time you might find that during each waking moment you are thinking about running and the race constantly. At the end of your training you are totally conditioned and prepared and when race day arrives you know that all the preparation has been worth it.

If you compare this to a diet, you will see that when you go on a diet, you have an end result in mind, which is similar to that race. Your goal is to reach a target weight or, to fit into a particular article of clothing. When you begin you might eliminate certain foods and be forced to learn about new foods and meals. This requires a considerable amount of effort and focus on food and eating - how to prepare it and in what quantities. Some diets have different tools to help you figure all this out and will assign a special colour or number to the different types. You then go about mixing and matching to make up your meal plans for the days, weeks or months that you are to be on the diet. So like that race you begin to train and then condition yourself to focus on food almost 24/7. During this time you maintain your new eating program and probably lose weight.

Once you reach your target it is like coming to the end of the race and you return to your "normal" lifestyle, piling weight back on again, because the diet is only designed to lose weight and now you go back to eating whatever the heart desires.

During your diet you were really training and conditioning yourself to think of food 24/7 – type, colour, quantity and category - non-stop intense focus on food. So now you are conditioned to focus on food all of the time and, with all restrictions and limitations over, this is a dangerous combination and the reason that so many people regain even more weight than they lost on the diet.

You can rest assured that this program is not a diet. It actually involves conditioning your mind with simple rules and behaviors which get in touch with your original program of eating to live, rather than living to eat. This is a sustainable lifestyle change and it becomes your permanent programming.

The Eight Rules For Successful Weight Loss Following 'Sheila Granger's Virtual Gastric Band'

There are just a few guidelines that you need to adhere to when learning to re-program your eating behavior. This whole concept of simple and effective change requires consistency. Repetition becomes habit and habits are what determine who we are. We are destined to fall back to the level of our conditioning and the Virtual Gastric Band will condition you for a healthy lifestyle.

The guidelines in this workbook are behaviors that have been adopted by fit and healthy people. While there are usually underlying causes for your inability to follow through your intentions, it is not the purpose of this short workbook to provide you with the tools to change your emotional responses as very few people are able to do that on their own. However, I want to tell you that it is possible to do this on your own – just do not give up.

If you have experienced the Virtual Gastric Band under hypnosis, then your stomach has been shrunk to the size of a golf ball and this workbook will increase the psychological impact of your Virtual Gastric Band, helping you to change your relationship with food.

Resolve now to take responsibility and follow these instructions to the letter - success will be yours.

Sheila Granger & Marc Carlin

"Any transition serious enough to alter your definition of self, will require not just small adjustments in your way of living and thinking, but a full-on metamorphosis"

~ Martha beck ~

Rule 1

BUY SOMETHING NEW

One very powerful psychological technique that I will be using is called the law of concentrated attention. Basically, if there is something in life that you really want – then behave as though you already have it – and you are very likely to get it.

Go out at your earliest opportunity and purchase an item of clothing in the size you want to be. It has to be something brand new and NOT something that you already have from your past which no longer fits - it need not be expensive. When you have bought it, hang it on the OUTSIDE of your wardrobe or in a place where you will see it often.

"The key to change... is to let go of fear."
~ Rosanne Cash ~

Rule #2

LISTEN TO THE CD

If you have gone through the Virtual Gastric Band program you will have been provided with a CD to listen to each day. Your practitioner will have advised you on the best time to listen.

The CD utilizes a multitude of the latest mind management techniques and is a very important part of your weight loss process. It is absolutely essential that you listen to it at least once a day (more if you can) for the next 28 days. The CD creates neural pathways in your brain regarding your association and attitude towards food. It also reinforces your weekly sessions.

The CD increases the effect tenfold and if you listen to it using stereo headphones via your MP3 player, you need to sit in a comfortable chair with both feet resting on the floor.

If you are reading this workbook to implement this program on your own, you can make your own recordings. Here are some simple instructions on how to do that.

If you can get some background trance music for your recording, all the better, but you can make it without the music.

Speak slowly and rhythmically and instruct yourself to relax the muscles in your body. Starting with your head and moving all the way down to your toes, instruct your body to relax each muscle group in turn. Mention the groups as you move down your body and give yourself time to relax each muscle completely.

Once all the muscles in your body are fully relaxed, instruct your mind to relax by walking down a staircase as you count backwards from 10. When you get to number 1 you will be fully relaxed in both mind and body - ready to accept hypnotic suggestions.

Then add suggestions onto the recording which support your lifestyle changes and your new responses. Such as:

- I am happier on a smaller amount of food.
- A small amount of food is more than enough to satisfy me.
- As soon as I start eating I'm losing my appetite.
- I'm amazed at how a small amount of food is more than enough for me.
- I eat my food slowly.
- I chew my food well.
- I eat my food slowly to taste every flavor

You can repeat these suggestions 3-10 times and when you are done you can imagine walking back up the stairs. As you count back up from 1-10 you become more alert, awakening totally at the count of 1, with your eyes open and wide awake.

Make your recording about fifteen minutes or so and then listen to it everyday at least once in the morning and then again when you get home from work - repetition reinforces the messages to your brain.

There are some more instructions on using trance through self-hypnosis towards the end of this workbook.

IMPORTANT – NEVER USE THE CD WHILE DRIVING OR OPERATING MACHINERY.

Your own recordings can include a number of positive statements about your new behaviors and will aid your weight loss. These recordings can last anywhere from five minutes to one hour. I would recommend you make affirmations at least five minutes and fifteen to thirty minutes for trance recordings.

"Nobody can go back and start a new beginning, but anyone can start today and make a new ending"
~ Maria Robinson ~

Rule #3

EAT SLOWLY AND CONSCIOUSLY

Eating is not a race. You are not working against the clock and there are no rewards for finishing quickly. When you eat you need to learn how to eat consciously without distractions. Many overweight people tell me they love food, but if your taste buds are in the mouth, why rush to get food into the stomach and away from sense of taste? The truth is that most people are not eating for pleasure. Nor are they really enjoying it, this is the just the minds way of rationalizing the process of overeating.

You can enjoy every mouthful of food, but slow your eating down and chew thoroughly at least 15-20 times per mouthful. An effective technique to help you eat slower is to put your knife and fork down between mouthfuls and if you are eating finger food or sandwiches put down the plate between mouthfuls. Even if your sandwich falls apart, that is perfectly fine. It will take you a bit more time to rebuild the sandwich before your next bite.

Do not eat in front of the television, computer or while reading as you will not be conscious of what you are putting in your mouth. Also keep any conversation friendly and upbeat.

Avoid emotionally charged situations while you are eating as this will hamper your ability to digest food properly.

Find a place where you can sit down and focus purely on the food in front of you. Make it so you only feel comfortable eating when you are sitting in a special place that you have reserved just for the purpose of eating. This is pretty easy when you are at home.

"There is nothing wrong with change, if it is in the right direction"
~ Winston Churchill ~

Rule #4

STOP EATING AS SOON AS YOU FEEL COMFORTABLE

Begin to get a sense of what hunger and satiety feel like. Imagine a scale of hunger with 1 being not hungry at all and 10 being ravenous. Ideally you want to develop a sense of your hunger level between 4-6 and when you know how that feels, you can begin to associate that level with the "time to eat" signal and during eating notice the satisfied signal on the top end of the scale.

"Be the change you want to see in the world"
~ Mahatma Gandhi ~

Rule #5

EAT ONLY THREE SMALL MEALS A DAY

For most people this is ideal and you can start off figuring you are like most people. Eat just three small meals a day – no more and no less. We are all familiar with how too much food feels in the stomach and we cannot blame the fast food restaurants for this. Eating out usually costs you five times the amount it would cost to buy the same food to prepare yourself. So in order to justify the increased prices that you are charged in a restaurant, the hospitality industry figured they could give you vast quantities of food so you would feel that you got your moneys worth.

Your doctor, your drug company, your pharmacy, your surgeon, your hospital, your nurse, and everyone you will depend upon in the near future will all be getting their share as a result of the generosity of that restaurant.

Most restaurant portions and even some pre-packaged supermarket meals are triple the amount you need to feel satisfied i.e. the size of a bagel has increased in size three times in just 20 years. The same is true for many other foods today.

One of my clients revealed to me recently that when she was at her favorite restaurant she looked at the portion of the meal she was served and recognized that if she ate all of it, she would have let someone else determine what the correct amount of food would be for her. She felt much more satisfied when she took back control and decide for herself what the appropriate amount of food should be.

Choose proteins first, as you need 50 – 70 grams of protein per day. A trick to help you adjust to a new smaller meal size would be to start using a smaller plate. You can then easily finish off your meal and feel content without the need, worry or stress of the attraction of leftover food on your plate. You could also ask your restaurant to give you 1/3 the food they would normally give you and immediately just pack the rest in a doggy bag.

"If you don't direct your change, your change will direct you"
~ Sheila Granger ~

Rule #6

BUY AND TAKE SOME MULTIVITAMINS

If the amount of food you will now be eating is drastically reduced from what you are used to, you might want to ensure you are still getting all of the vitamins you need. Supplementing your dietary intake with some vitamins can be a good way to do that. You should check with someone that is knowledgeable in this area to help you decide. Also, when you embark on a weight loss journey you should consult with your physician to get their advice and guidelines on what would be appropriate for you.

This program in no way gives you any medical advice and you are taking responsibility for your own health.

"Change is the basis of living.
Be willing to let go of your definition of
'you' and begin the metamorphosis of what
you are destined to become"
~ Marc Carlin ~

Rule #7

DRINK PLENTY OF FLUIDS AND CHOOSE ONLY LOW CALORIE LIQUIDS

This primarily means water. Drink water in place of any and all other drinks you usually consume. I do not recommend any sugar-free or artificially sweetened drinks of any kind - just drink water.

It has often been reported that as we age, we exchange what we used to recognize as a signal of thirst for hunger and begin to eat when we should have just had some water. It is a great strategy to drink water before you eat anything and if it was just thirst, you will find you no longer want to eat. If after twenty minutes to a half an hour you still feel hungry, then it probably is real hunger and you can go ahead and have one of your three small meals.

" Things do not change; we change"
~ Henry David Thoreau ~

Rule #8

EXERCISE

Exercise is important for a number of reasons. One of those reasons is to build muscle which gives you strength and tone your body so you look and feel great. It is also thought that when you embark on a weight loss program, by reducing your fuel intake, you force your body to use the fuel you already have stored i.e. deposits of fat. Your body can, however, also take its fuel supply from your muscles leaving your body full of fat which is not a pretty picture.

One way to ignite your fat burning ability is to exercise regularly and this program encourages exercise. It is very important with the Virtual Gastric Band that you take up some form of exercise for at least thirty minutes per day. This can be going for a walk - you can just step out of your house and walk in one direction for about 15 minutes and then turn around and walk back. It makes no difference at this point what your ultimate goals are, but it is important to start increasing your level of activity now. If thirty minutes of exercise is too much for you at this point, then commit to five minutes. There is no valid reason to excuse yourself from consistently doing your five minutes each day - commit to this and get started.

When you embark on a weight loss journey you should consult your physician to get their advice and guidelines on what is appropriate for you. This program in no way gives you medical advice and you are taking responsibility for your own health.

As you will be eating less than your body needs to operate, it will burn up its reserves. If you do not exercise daily, your body will metabolize your unused muscle and you will lose muscle mass and strength. Exercise will communicate to your body that you want to use your muscles and force it to burn the fat instead. Walk, skip, and dance around the house – move.

Self Hypnosis

The Simple Secrets To Successful Self-Hypnosis

Easy techniques for successful transformation

"Your belief determines your action and your action determines your results, but first you have to believe." ~Mark Victor Hansen

Beginning The Process of Programming Your Mind

This is a simple program to direct your mind to receive the auto-suggestions of your choice. I have broken this process down into five easy to follow stages, that allow you to become familiar with the trance experience.

Give yourself time to process each stage, perhaps a couple of days, practicing each stage a number of times each day.

Stage 1

These simple but powerful techniques will benefit you as you integrate them into your lifestyle. It will take a commitment on your part, but I assure you, it is a small amount of your time, and well worth the investment.

This first stage is about relieving everyday stress. Depending on how much stress you might be feeling at the moment, you might find all of it dissipates, or most, or some. This is a simple method of relieving stress, and the more you do it, the better you will be at it, and the faster you see the results.

Read through the instructions and then practice doing the technique immediately afterwards. You can do this either sitting or standing. If you have a problem with keeping yourself balanced, find a place to sit down, or lean against the wall. Take a deep breath in, and as you breathe out, close your eyes and relax the muscles around the eyes until they are so relaxed that they will not work. As you do this, continue to focus on your rhythmic breathing. Once you are able relax your eye muscles, hold onto the relaxation for about sixty seconds and when you open your eyes, notice how much more relaxed, and in control you feel.

When should you do this? Anytime you want to take a break.

1. Weight Loss: If you are using this technique for weight loss, you can do it anytime you want to eat something you know would be better left on the plate, in the kitchen or, on the menu.

2. Stop Smoking: If you are using this for quitting smoking, you would use this technique anytime you feel the need for a cigarette.

3. Stress Reduction: Before and/or after any stressful situation.

Have fun practicing this exercise and do it as many times as you want to during the day. You cannot over do it, however, be safe in the area you choose to practice.

In your next stage, we will begin the process of using visualization in a unique, easy and fun way to program your mind through mental rehearsal. When you practice what it is that you want, your subconscious will go out of its way to make sure you get it.

Stage 2

"It isn't what you have, or who you are, or where you are, or what you are doing that makes you happy or unhappy.

It is what you think about."

~Dale Carnegie

If you have been practicing regularly, what you learned in Stage 1 for a couple of days, by now, you will be feeling relaxed and more comfortable.

We learn by trial and error and you are in the process of learning through your own experience.

So, if you have taken action, you are gaining experience and learning to relax as an act of will. If you had difficulty being relaxed in the past, you will soon be able to relax as you practice.

What we rehearse, we become accustomed to doing and mental rehearsal is just as important as physical rehearsal. In this second stage you learn how to mentally rehearse without having to put out much effort. This technique is to be done before you go to bed. It is simple, and easy to do, but like all of my techniques, it is extremely powerful.

Each night as you go to sleep say to yourself, *"every day, in every way, I am better, and better"*. This is an old phrase used by a hypnotist from the early part of the last century. This hypnotist, Emile Coué, traveled around the world educating people on the techniques of auto-suggestion.

For the really powerful part of this process I want you to bring up a picture in your mind of whatever it is that you want to accomplish. If it is losing weight, bring up an image of yourself doing one particular behavior that will result in you losing weight, such as, eating small amounts of food. If you want to stop smoking, bring up an image of yourself taking in deep breaths of fresh air feeling a wonderful sense of control. Make this image a motion picture and see it in your minds eye as you repeat that phrase ten times to yourself.

"Every day in every way, I'm better, and better, and better."

As your subconscious mind does not sleep, you have just programmed it to do a mental rehearsal all night long.

In the next stage you will learn how to go into the hypnotic trance state on command. You will also learn the secret of creating powerful suggestions to make your subconscious do what it is you want it to do.

Stage 3

"Do not wait; the time will never be "just right." Start where you stand, and work with whatever tools you may have at your command, and better tools will be found as you go along."

~Napoleon Hill

Before we get to Stage 3 I would like to review what you have learned and practiced so far.

In Stage 1 you learned a really simple technique for getting relaxed at will. You are no longer at the mercy of the things going on outside of you. You can be concerned, able to respond in a satisfactory way, but you do not have to stress out about it - because you now have a tool for de-stressing.

In Stage 2 you learned to use the power of your subconscious whilst sleeping to practice the behaviors and responses you want to become your conditioned responses.

Now we are onto the process of teaching you how to go into a hypnotic trance on demand and how to give yourself suggestions for change.

1) Continue doing Stage 1, the relaxation on command when necessary and Stage 2, the pre-sleep technique you already learned.

2) In addition sit in a comfortable chair with your back and head supported.

3) Focus your eyes on a spot opposite you, slightly above eye level, about 45 degrees up. It could be a spot on the wall high up, or the corner of a picture frame for example.

4) Take three deep breaths. Hold the third breath for the mental count of three and as you let it go with a sigh, close your eyes and feel your whole body relaxing even more.

RELAX and allow yourself to fall into a deep hypnotic rest. As you relax in your seat, feel your breathing regulate and slow down.

Now imagine yourself on the top of a staircase with ten steps. As you walk slowly down each step, think to yourself the words *"deeper and deeper"*. Use your imagination and really start to feel yourself going down the stairs and continue to think to yourself *"deeper and deeper"*.

By reaching the bottom step, you have become so very relaxed and calm you will now be in your hypnotic state.

Remain in this state for as long as you can be comfortable. Make it about five to ten minutes to start allowing your mind to wander.

When you are ready to emerge from trance, count upwards from 1-5, imagining with each count that you feel more vibrant and energized. Think to yourself, *"I feel better mentally, physically, and emotionally"*.

By practicing this technique, you are making it easier and easier for you to access this level of relaxation. Your mind and body are practicing relaxing in unison and this ability to go into this very relaxed state, both mentally and physically, becomes easier and quicker for you to achieve.

Stage 4

"Not to have control over the senses is like sailing in a rudderless ship, bound to break to pieces on coming in contact with the very first rock."

~Mohandas Karamchand Gandhi

I trust you have become better at guiding yourself into trance, relaxing at will and allowing yourself to accept the positive suggestions for the changes you want to make.

This is Stage 4 of this 5 stage process of learning self-hypnosis. In Stage 1, you learned a really simple technique on how to relax at will. You are no longer at the mercy of the things going on outside of you. You can be concerned, able to respond in a satisfactory way, but you do not become stressed because you now have a tool to de-stress.

In Stage 2, you learned a way to do mental rehearsal without putting out much effort. By using the power of your subconscious whilst sleeping, you have practiced the behaviors and responses that you want to become your conditioned responses.

In Stage 3, you learned how to guide yourself into a deeply relaxed state. This is the first level of hypnosis. The first level of hypnosis is enough to begin behavior pattern changes through auto-suggestion.

Now we are onto the process of teaching yourself how to go into hypnosis on command and how to give yourself suggestions for change.

The more you practice self-hypnosis, the better you will become at it. You will soon realize that you can achieve not only a deeper level of relaxation but you will also be able to achieve it faster.

Giving yourself auto-suggestion

1) Figure out what it is that you want to accomplish. Is it a change of habit, a behavior or thought?

Whatever it is, have a clear image of what the outcome will be like. This can be what it is that you will look like, what your behavior will be like, what you will feel like, etc. You can use that image, or if you have trouble holding onto the picture, you can connect a key word to that image that represents that visual to you.

This will be your prepared thoughts that you use when you reach your level of self-hypnosis.

2) Get yourself deeply relaxed to the first level of hypnosis.

3) Once you reach the last step and feel completely relaxed, test your eye closure. Tell yourself in your mind that you can not open your eyes, they are shut tight. After you test them and cannot open them, stop and continue to relax.

4) Now, you are ready to give yourself auto-suggestions.

The auto-suggestion will be the image or keyword(s) you have previously chosen. See your image or keyword(s) over and over, vividly in your mind's eye.

For each new goal do this exercise at least twenty-one days in a row then continue for reinforcement. Be patient and you WILL achieve your results. and continue to relax.

Stage 5

"Great works are performed not by strength but by perseverance."

~Samuel Johnson

Now that you have the techniques to affect powerful change from the inside out, this stage will give you examples of how to formulate suggestions for the most common complaints people see me for.

Now that you have gotten even better at going into trance, reducing stress, and relaxing on cue, I am going to teach you the fundamentals of creating suggestions for change.

In Stage 1, you learned a really simple technique on how to relax at will. You are no longer at the mercy of the things going on outside of you. You can be concerned, able to respond in a satisfactory way, but you do not have to stress out about it because you now have a tool to de-stress.

In Stage 2 you learned a way to do mental rehearsal without much effort. By using the power of your subconscious, while you are sleeping, you have practiced the behaviors and responses that you want to become your conditioned responses.

In Stage 3 you learned how to guide yourself into a deeply relaxed state. This is the first level of hypnosis and is enough to begin behavior pattern changes through auto-suggestion.

In Stage 4 you learned how to go into hypnosis on demand, and how to give yourself suggestions for change.

Now, in this 5th Stage, I am going to show you how to formulate suggestions before going into trance, so you can program your mind to achieve that goal.

Suggestion is how you specify what your goals are and then give your subconscious specific instructions to get those goals. This puts your conscious and subconscious mind on the same page - once that happens, you are almost guaranteed success.

When formulating suggestions for self-hypnosis, you want to be specific about what you want as an outcome. You might have heard the expression *"be careful of what you wish for"*. I think this came about because of the focus on outcomes instead of the desired effect is. For example, if you give yourself a suggestion for attracting lots of money and do not make it very specific, you might get money as a result of some kind of insurance windfall because of a tragedy. This would probably not be what you want.

If you were wanting to lose weight and that was all that you focused on, that could lead to you losing weight through harmful ways, which would most assuredly not be what you want. In the movie *The Devil Wears Prada*, I remember one of the main characters saying excitedly, *"I'm just one stomach virus away from goal weight!"* – I thought that was funny, but not a desirable thing to program yourself for.

So be specific in the formulation of your suggestions and add a benefit that you will get when you follow the suggestion.

And as promised, here are some suggestions you can give

yourself for weight loss:

"I enjoy eating healthy food and my body feels good when I do"

"I eat slowly and get to taste my food fully"

"The healthiest foods taste the best to me"

"I exercise daily and feel invigorated when I do"

"When I exercise daily, I get a sense of accomplishment and confidence that stays with me all day"

When you give yourself these suggestions, bring up an image of you behaving as the suggestion suggests.

The following images are specifically for the Virtual Gastric Band process and can be used in conjunction with the previous suggestions for weight loss:

Imagine your stomach shrinking down smaller and smaller until it is the size of a golf ball.

Imagine your stomach so very small that it can only accept a very small amount of food.

Imagine that stomach now so very small because of the restrictions of a band around the top of it.

Imagine how your appetite has become so very stifled and how just a small amount of food is more than enough to satisfy you.

Imagine how tight your stomach feels.

Imagine how such a small amount of food satisfies you.

Imagine eating slowly, enjoying each small mouthful.
Auto suggestions for Smoking Cessation would be as
follows:

"I am a non-smoker and I have more time to do the
things I want to do"

"I am a non-smoker and my lungs feel better breathing
fresh clean air"

"I am a non-smoker and I feel calmer and more in
control"

"I am a non-smoker and my clothes smell fresh, my hands
smell fresh, my hair smells fresh, my breath smells fresh"

"I am a non-smoker and people accept me more easily"

"I am a non-smoker and I breathe more easily and I am
more calm"

Enjoy practicing these techniques for powerful permanent and
profound change.

Many thanks,

Sheila Granger and Marc Carlin

Keeping Track

Weekly Statistics - 1

Week Starting Date _____

Weight: _____

Neck Size: _____

Chest Size: _____

Waist Size: _____

Hip Size: _____

Left Thigh Size: _____

Right Thigh Size: _____

Recommended calories per day for
height, weight, age and gender _____

Recommended weight for height, age and gender _____

Current Weight: _____
Target Permanent Weight: _____
Fat to release: _____
Number of weeks to Target Permanent Weight =
(pounds / 1.5)= _____
Target Date to Reach My Goal: _____

Date: _____

Time	Amount	Food Selection	Hunger rating	Mood

Water								

Successes for Today

Date: _____

Time	Amount	Food Selection	Hunger rating	Mood

Water									

Successes for Today

Date: _____

Time	Amount	Food Selection	Hunger rating	Mood

Water									

Successes for Today

Date: _____

Time	Amount	Food Selection	Hunger rating	Mood

Water									

Successes for Today

Date: _____

Time	Amount	Food Selection	Hunger rating	Mood

Water									

Successes for Today

Date: _____

Time	Amount	Food Selection	Hunger rating	Mood

Water									

Successes for Today

Date: _____

Time	Amount	Food Selection	Hunger rating	Mood

Water								

Successes for Today

Weekly Statistics - 2

Week Starting Date _____

Weight: _____

Neck Size: _____

Chest Size: _____

Waist Size: _____

Hip Size: _____

Left Thigh Size: _____

Right Thigh Size: _____

Recommended calories per day for
height, weight, age and gender _____

Recommended weight for height, age and gender _____

Current Weight: _____
Target Permanent Weight: _____
Fat to release: _____
Number of weeks to Target Permanent Weight =
(pounds / 1.5)= _____
Target Date to Reach My Goal: _____

Sheila Granger & Marc Carlin

Date: _____

Time	Amount	Food Selection	Hunger rating	Mood

Water									

Successes for Today

Date: _____

Time	Amount	Food Selection	Hunger rating	Mood

Water								

Successes for Today

Date: _____

Time	Amount	Food Selection	Hunger rating	Mood

Water								

Successes for Today

Date: _____

Time	Amount	Food Selection	Hunger rating	Mood

Water								

Successes for Today

Date: _____

Time	Amount	Food Selection	Hunger rating	Mood

Water									

Successes for Today

Date: _____

Time	Amount	Food Selection	Hunger rating	Mood

Water								

Successes for Today

Date: _____

Time	Amount	Food Selection	Hunger rating	Mood

Water									

Successes for Today

Weekly Statistics - 3

Week Starting Date _____

Weight: _____

Neck Size: _____

Chest Size: _____

Waist Size: _____

Hip Size: _____

Left Thigh Size: _____

Right Thigh Size: _____

Recommended calories per day for
height, weight, age and gender _____

Recommended weight for height, age and gender _____

Current Weight: _____
Target Permanent Weight: _____
Fat to release: _____
Number of weeks to Target Permanent Weight =
(pounds / 1.5)= _____
Target Date to Reach My Goal: _____

Date: _____

Time	Amount	Food Selection	Hunger rating	Mood

Water									

Successes for Today

Date: _____

Time	Amount	Food Selection	Hunger rating	Mood

Water								

Successes for Today

Date: _____

Time	Amount	Food Selection	Hunger rating	Mood

Water									

Successes for Today

Date: _____

Time	Amount	Food Selection	Hunger rating	Mood

Water									

Successes for Today

Date: _____

Time	Amount	Food Selection	Hunger rating	Mood

Water									

Successes for Today

Date: _____

Time	Amount	Food Selection	Hunger rating	Mood

Water									

Successes for Today

Date: _____

Time	Amount	Food Selection	Hunger rating	Mood

Water								

Successes for Today

Weekly Statistics - 4

Week Starting Date _____

Weight: _____

Neck Size: _____

Chest Size: _____

Waist Size: _____

Hip Size: _____

Left Thigh Size: _____

Right Thigh Size: _____

Recommended calories per day for
height, weight, age and gender _____

Recommended weight for height, age and gender _____

Current Weight: _____
Target Permanent Weight: _____
Fat to release: _____
Number of weeks to Target Permanent Weight =
(pounds / 1.5)= _____
Target Date to Reach My Goal: _____

.

Date: _____

Time	Amount	Food Selection	Hunger rating	Mood

Water								

Successes for Today

Date: _____

Time	Amount	Food Selection	Hunger rating	Mood

Water									

Successes for Today

Date: _____

Time	Amount	Food Selection	Hunger rating	Mood

Water								

Successes for Today

Date: _____

Time	Amount	Food Selection	Hunger rating	Mood

Water									

Successes for Today

Date: _____

Time	Amount	Food Selection	Hunger rating	Mood

Water									

Successes for Today

Date: _____

Time	Amount	Food Selection	Hunger rating	Mood

Water								

Successes for Today

Date: _____

Time	Amount	Food Selection	Hunger rating	Mood

Water									

Successes for Today

Weekly Statistics - 5

Week Starting Date _____

Weight: _____

Neck Size: _____

Chest Size: _____

Waist Size: _____

Hip Size: _____

Left Thigh Size: _____

Right Thigh Size: _____

Recommended calories per day for
height, weight, age and gender _____

Recommended weight for height, age and gender _____

Current Weight: _____
Target Permanent Weight: _____
Fat to release: _____
Number of weeks to Target Permanent Weight =
(pounds / 1.5)= _____
Target Date to Reach My Goal: _____

Date: _____

Time	Amount	Food Selection	Hunger rating	Mood

Water									

Successes for Today

Date: _____

Time	Amount	Food Selection	Hunger rating	Mood

Water								

Successes for Today

Date: _____

Time	Amount	Food Selection	Hunger rating	Mood

Water									

Successes for Today

Date: _____

Time	Amount	Food Selection	Hunger rating	Mood

Water								

Successes for Today

Date: _____

Time	Amount	Food Selection	Hunger rating	Mood

Water									

Successes for Today

Date: _____

Time	Amount	Food Selection	Hunger rating	Mood

Water								

Successes for Today

Date: _____

Time	Amount	Food Selection	Hunger rating	Mood

Water								

Successes for Today

Weekly Statistics - 6

Week Starting Date _____

Weight: _____

Neck Size: _____

Chest Size: _____

Waist Size: _____

Hip Size: _____

Left Thigh Size: _____

Right Thigh Size: _____

Recommended calories per day for
height, weight, age and gender _____

Recommended weight for height, age and gender _____

Current Weight: _____
Target Permanent Weight: _____
Fat to release: _____
Number of weeks to Target Permanent Weight =
(pounds / 1.5)= _____
Target Date to Reach My Goal: _____

Date: _____

Time	Amount	Food Selection	Hunger rating	Mood

Water									

Successes for Today

Date: _____

Time	Amount	Food Selection	Hunger rating	Mood

Water									

Successes for Today

Date: _____

Time	Amount	Food Selection	Hunger rating	Mood

Water									

Successes for Today

Date: _____

Time	Amount	Food Selection	Hunger rating	Mood

Water									

Successes for Today

Date: _____

Time	Amount	Food Selection	Hunger rating	Mood

Water								

Successes for Today

Date: _____

Time	Amount	Food Selection	Hunger rating	Mood

Water								

Successes for Today

Date: _____

Time	Amount	Food Selection	Hunger rating	Mood

Water								

Successes for Today

ACKNOWLEDGMENTS

I am fortunate enough to be surrounded by a fantastic network of like-minded people who believe in me and know that anything is possible if you just set your mind to it. The people at Inception House Publishing who made this book happen. Marc Carlin, my co-author and training associate in the US. UK medical professionals who recognize the power of hypnotherapy, as a tool to combat many ailments and medical conditions that drain the public purse. The UK press for spreading the word about a potential solution to the worldwide obesity epidemic. My teacher, Brian Glenn, whose initial training and support has benefitted me. My parents for always being there. Jenny for providing the gift of motherhood. Judy for keeping me grounded. Stuart, for running my bath and making my dinner. My PR agents, Jess and Leigh Clark who believed in my work and helped me promote it. The women and men from around the world who have wanted to help themselves and make a positive change in their lives, and who have all made a difference in mine. My dependable and loving friends who celebrate with me. To everyone who has left a lasting impression. The mind, for it's infinite power.

~Sheila

I originally wanted to acknowledge all the previous generations that came before me because in life, everything that we've experienced becomes a part of who we are and what we allow ourselves to achieve. But on re-thinking things I decided to get to the nitty gritty of those who directly contributed to my success in this field and in writing this book. Sheila Granger, the developer of this program and my co-author obviously has played a significant role in this process. My friends and mentors in the hypnosis field, Mark Cunningham who gave me a solid understanding of the hypnosis ritual along with the ways to most effectively hook people into the changes they so yearn for. Cal Banyan, who taught me how to use the hypnotic process in a systematic way. Barry Seedman who first showed me hypnosis at work and sparked a burning passion in me to seek out how to use this age old profession to help many. To George Bien, who gave me my first verifiable trance experience. Don Mottin, Jerry Kein, Gil Boyne, Ormond McGill, Dave Elman, and countless other hypnotists they learned from. And all my clients, because in my world every interaction is a learning experience. Thank you all.

~Marc

Resources

Sheila Granger's Virtual Gastric Band Practitioners

This book presents the strategies and guidelines that we offer our clients who come to visit us for help in reclaiming their proper shape and size. The true benefit of our program comes from the result of combining this process with hypnotic technique. And the best way to learn the proper way of using your mind is by working with a consulting hypnotist or hypnotherapist.

You can get more information about working with Sheila Granger, UK Clinical Hypnotherapist at:
  http://SheilaGranger.com

You can get more information about working with Marc Carlin, Consulting Hypnotist at:
  http://www.HypnoticState.com

We have also spent the last year training other hypnotists and hypnotherapists around the world in the techniques of Sheila Granger's Virtual Gastric Band. You can find one of our practioners in your area to work with at:
  http://VirtualGastricBand.net

If you yourself would like to train to become a practitioner of Sheila Granger's Virtual Gastric Band you can get more information about our live trainings at:
  http://VirtualGastricBandTraining.com

Made in the USA
Middletown, DE
29 January 2015